# The

# Hashimotos cookbook

Nourishing Recipes for Thyroid Wellness
on the AIP disorder

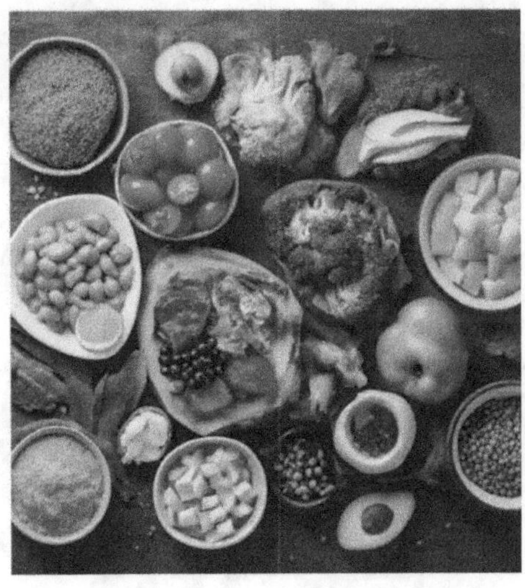

**Linda A. Ivey**

**GAIN ACCESS TO MORE BOOKS FROM ME**

**THANK YOU FOR CHOOSING US.**

**We Appreciate Your Kind Support And We Hope
You Got Something Out Of It.**

**If You Enjoy This Book, It Will Be Great To Leave a
Review On Amazon . It Means a Lot To Us.**

*To all the men and women who is striving to live
well with Hashimotos disease and other
autoimmune conditions*

# Contents

# Introduction

## Understanding Hashimoto's: A Brief Overview

**H**ashimoto's thyroiditis, named after the Japanese physician who first described it in 1912, is an autoimmune disorder that affects the thyroid gland. This condition occurs when the immune system mistakenly recognizes the thyroid as a threat and begins to attack it, leading to inflammation and damage.

In this section, we delve into the fundamental aspects of Hashimoto's, providing readers with a clear understanding of the condition:

1. **The Thyroid: A Vital Player**
   - Explore the crucial role of the thyroid gland in regulating metabolism and overall health.
   - Understand how thyroid hormones influence various bodily functions.
2. **Unraveling Autoimmunity**
   - Gain insights into the concept of autoimmune diseases and how the

immune system's misguided response triggers Hashimoto's.

- Learn about the specific antibodies involved in the attack on the thyroid.

3. **Common Signs and Symptoms**

- Identify the typical indicators of Hashimoto's, ranging from fatigue and weight gain to changes in mood and skin issues.
- Recognize the importance of early detection and seeking medical advice for timely intervention.

4. **Diagnostic Process**

- Navigate through the diagnostic journey, from initial symptoms to blood tests and thyroid function assessments.
- Understand the significance of TSH, T4, and T3 levels in the diagnostic process.

5. **Risk Factors and Triggers**

- Explore the factors that may contribute to the development of Hashimoto's, including genetic predisposition and environmental triggers.
- Gain insights into lifestyle choices that can influence the course of the condition.

### 6. Living with Hashimoto's: A Holistic Perspective

- Emphasize the need for a comprehensive approach to managing Hashimoto's, including medical interventions, dietary changes, and lifestyle adjustments.
- Highlight the importance of regular monitoring and communication with healthcare professionals.

## Importance of Nutrition in Managing Hashimoto's

To effectively treat Hashimoto's thyroiditis, a disorder in which the immune system attacks and destroys the thyroid gland, proper nutrition is essential. Making thoughtful and educated food choices may improve thyroid function, reduce symptoms, and enhance general well-being. This section delves into the critical impact that diet plays in managing Hashimoto's disease.

### 1. Boosting Thyroid Activity

Recognize the nutrients—such as zinc, selenium, and iodine—that are necessary for the thyroid to operate at its best.

Examine how a balanced diet might provide the components required for the synthesis of thyroid hormones.

## 2. Reducing Inflammation with Anti-Inflammatory Diet

Choose and include anti-inflammatory foods to help lessen thyroid inflammation and the autoimmune reaction.

Find out how antioxidants, phytonutrients, and omega-3 fatty acids support a healthy immune system.

## 3. Achieving Blood Sugar Equilibrium

Understand the link between blood sugar abnormalities and Hashimoto's disease.

Examine how a well-balanced diet rich in fiber, complex carbs, and modest amounts of protein may help to stabilize blood sugar levels.

## 4. Autoimmunity and Gut Health

Examine the connection between autoimmune diseases like Hashimoto's and intestinal health.

Find out how a gut-friendly diet, probiotics, and prebiotics may help maintain a healthy digestive tract and perhaps even reduce symptoms.

### 5. The Effects of Dairy and Gluten

Examine the connection between dairy, gluten, and Hashimoto's.

Recognize the possible advantages of a dairy- and gluten-free diet in lowering inflammation and alleviating symptoms in some people.

### 6. Using Supplements of Nutrients Strategically

Talk about how specific vitamin supplements may help with deficiencies that are often linked to Hashimoto's disease.

Stress the need to consult with medical specialists to identify each patient's unique supplement requirements.

### 7. Tailoring the Diet for Hashimoto's

Recognize that every person's reaction to dietary modifications is different.

To find trigger foods, encourage experimenting with elimination diets and gradual reintroduction.

### 8. Synergy between nutrition and lifestyle factors

Emphasize how diet and lifestyle choices, such as getting enough sleep, managing stress, and exercising often, work together to promote overall well-being.

# The Hashimoto's Journey

## Personal Story of Triumph

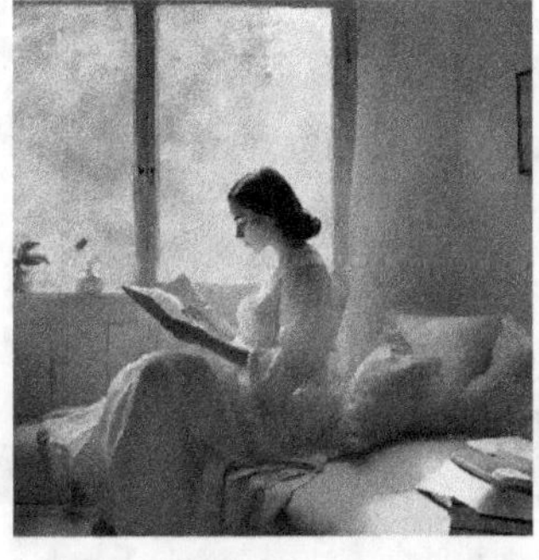

Meet Lisa, a resilient and spirited woman whose life took an unexpected turn when she was diagnosed with Hashimoto's thyroiditis. Lisa's journey is a testament to the power of determination, adaptability, and the transformative impact of holistic self-care.

Lisa's story begins with the subtle onset of symptoms—fatigue that seemed to deepen with each passing day, unexplained weight gain, and a persistent fog that clouded her once-vibrant mind. It took numerous visits to different healthcare professionals before Lisa received the diagnosis that would reshape her life.

Upon learning about her Hashimoto's diagnosis, Lisa embarked on a journey of self-discovery and empowerment. Determined not to be defined by her condition, she embraced a proactive approach to managing her health. Lisa dove into extensive research, and came across **"the hashimotos cookbook"** arming herself with knowledge about the intricate connection between nutrition, lifestyle, and Hashimoto's.

Lisa's kitchen transformed into a haven of healing, where she experimented with thyroid-friendly recipes, embracing nutrient-dense foods and eliminating potential triggers. Whole grains, lean proteins, and a colorful array of fruits and vegetables became the cornerstone of her daily meals. Lisa also discovered the art of mindful eating, savoring each bite as a gesture of self-love and nourishment.

Beyond the kitchen, Lisa incorporated stress-relief practices into her daily routine. Yoga and meditation became anchors in her life, helping to calm the autoimmune storm within. She recognized the importance of quality sleep and prioritized rest as a non-negotiable element of her healing journey.

Lisa's journey was not without challenges. There were moments of frustration and setbacks, but each obstacle fueled her determination to regain control over her life. Regular check-ins with her healthcare team ensured that she was on the right track, and adjustments were made as needed.

Over time, Lisa began to experience a positive transformation. Her energy levels increased, the persistent brain fog lifted, and she felt a renewed sense of vitality. Lisa's journey was not just about managing her Hashimoto's; it was about reclaiming her life and rediscovering her true self.

**Today**, Lisa is not just a survivor; she is a thriver. Her story serves as an inspiration to others facing the challenges of autoimmune conditions. Lisa's journey reminds us that with knowledge, resilience, and a holistic approach to well-being, it is possible to not only endure but to flourish in the face of adversity.

# Chapter 1

# Building a Thyroid-Friendly Kitchen

## Stocking Your Pantry with Essentials

The first step in developing a kitchen that is conducive to thyroid health is to carefully fill your pantry with key items that are beneficial to the treatment of Hashimoto's thyroid condition. If you make the proper decisions, you can improve your diet, reduce inflammation, and take steps toward improving your overall health. The following is an exhaustive list of items that should be maintained in your pantry:

1. **Whole Grains:**
   - Instead, choose whole grains that are high in nutrients, such as quinoa, brown rice, and oats that are gluten-free.
   - These grains are a source of critical vitamins, minerals, and fiber, and they do

not cause any possible allergies to be triggered.

2. **The legumes:**
   - A wide range of legumes, including chickpeas, lentils, and black beans, should be included in the diet.
   - Legumes include plant-based protein, fiber, and a spectrum of minerals helpful for thyroid health.

3. **Healthy Fats:**
   - Make sure to consume foods that contain healthy fats, such as olive oil, avocados, almonds, and seeds.
   - Omega-3 fatty acids, found in walnuts and flaxseeds, may have anti-inflammatory benefits.

4. **The Sources of Protein:**
   - Incorporate lean protein sources such as chicken, fish, eggs, and plant-based choices like tofu and tempeh.
   - Adequate protein is necessary for thyroid function and general muscular health.

5. **Gluten-Free Flours:**
   - Explore gluten-free flours such as almond flour, coconut flour, and cassava flour.

- These substitutes may be utilized in baking and cooking, catering to persons with gluten intolerance.

6. **Dairy Alternatives:**
   - Opt for dairy substitutes like almond milk, coconut milk, or hemp milk.
   - Some persons with Hashimoto's may prefer to forgo dairy owing to its possible inflammatory effects.

7. **Fresh Produce:**
   - Prioritize a colorful variety of fruits and vegetables rich in antioxidants and critical minerals.
   - Include seasonal and organic choices wherever available.

8. **Herbs and Spices:**
   - Build a collection of herbs and spices such as turmeric, ginger, and cilantro.
   - These components not only provide taste but also have anti-inflammatory and antioxidant benefits.

9. **Canned Goods:**
   - Keep canned products like chopped tomatoes, beans, and fish for simple meal preparation.

- Choose BPA-free cans and check labels for additional preservatives.

## 10. Seeds and Nuts:
- Include seeds like chia, flax, and pumpkin seeds, as well as a range of nuts.
- These are wonderful providers of healthy fats, protein, and important minerals.

## 11. Gluten-Free Pasta and Grains:
- Explore gluten-free pasta alternatives made from rice, quinoa, or lentils.
- Have a range of gluten-free grains like millet and sorghum for different meal alternatives.

## 12. Low-Sugar Sweeteners:
- Choose natural sweeteners such as honey, maple syrup, or stevia.
- Limit refined sugars and artificial sweeteners, since they may alter blood sugar and inflammatory levels.

## 13. Culinary Basics:

Stock up on essentials like sea salt, black pepper, and high-quality vinegar for flavoring foods.

Consider using Himalayan or iodized salt to support iodine intake.

## 14. Teas and Infusions:

Incorporate herbal teas like chamomile, peppermint, and ginger for their calming effects.

These drinks may be part of a thoughtful and hydrated habit.

Remember to frequently examine and rotate products in your pantry to guarantee freshness. Tailoring your pantry to meet your specific requirements and tastes is a critical component of effectively treating Hashimoto's via a well-rounded and nutritionally supportive strategy.

## Kitchen Tools for Effortless Cooking

Setting up a thyroid-friendly kitchen entails not just stocking the necessary materials but also having the required equipment to make your cooking experience quick and pleasurable. Here's a list of basic kitchen products that will help you cook healthful meals while managing Hashimoto's:

- **High-Quality Blender:**

Invest in a strong blender for smoothies, soups, and sauces. It's a flexible tool for introducing nutrient-dense items into your diet.

- **Food Processor:**

A food processor is good for chopping, slicing, and shredding vegetables and nuts. It saves time and effort in meal preparation.

- **Quality Knives:**

A set of sharp, high-quality knives is crucial for accuracy in chopping fruits, vegetables, and meats. Properly chopped components guarantee consistent cooking and excellent appearance.

- **Slow Cooker or Instant Pot:**

These culinary devices are a time-saving blessing. They enable for simple and gradual cooking of stews, soups, and cereals, conserving nutrients and tastes.

- **Spiralizer:**

Create vegetable noodles using a spiralizer to integrate more vegetables into your diet. Zucchini, sweet potatoes, and carrots all be made into delightful alternatives to classic spaghetti.

- **Steamer Basket:**

A steamer basket maintains the nutritious elements of vegetables. It's a fast and nutritious cooking technique that keeps the bright colors and textures of your food.

- **Cast Iron Skillet:**

A cast iron pan is wonderful for uniform cooking and is a good source of dietary iron. It's flexible, and resilient, and improves the taste of your foods.

- **Non-Stick Baking Mats and Pans:**

Opt for non-stick surfaces to eliminate the need for unnecessary cooking oils. Silicone baking mats and pans are simple to clean and lessen the chance of sticking.

- **Measuring Cups and Spoons:**

Accurate measurements are vital, particularly when following strict dietary requirements. Invest in a set of trustworthy measuring cups and spoons.

- **Food Scale:**

A food scale is important for accurate portion control and measuring ingredients, particularly if you're managing certain dietary needs.

- **Glass Storage Containers:**

Store  leftovers and meal preps in glass containers to minimize any chemical leaching from plastic. Glass containers are also microwave-safe and simple to clean.

- **Collapsible Colander:**

Save room in your kitchen with a foldable colander. It's excellent for draining spaghetti, cleaning veggies, and convenient storing.

- **Herb Mill or Mincer:**

Fresh herbs offer a taste without extra salt. A herb mill or mincer makes it simple to include these fragrant herbs in your dishes.

- **Quality Cutting Boards:**

Invest in cutting boards made of bamboo or other sustainable materials. Having different boards helps you to segregate ingredients and prevent cross-contamination.

- **Nut Milk Bag or Cheesecloth:**

If you create your own nut milk or strain liquids, a nut milk bag or cheesecloth is a valuable tool for producing smooth and pulp-free results.

# Chapter 2

# Breakfast Boosters

## Energizing Smoothie Bowls

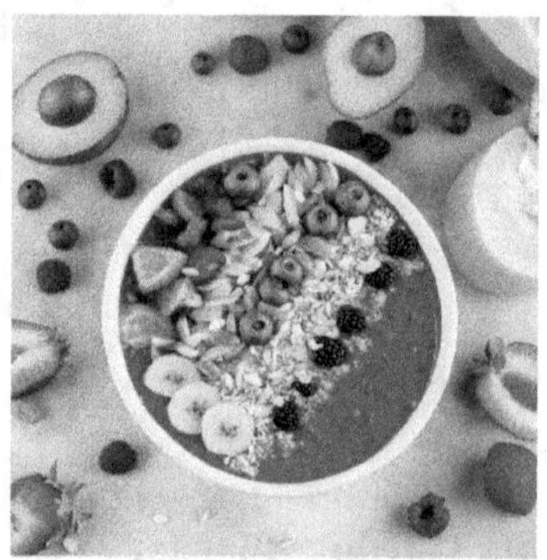

**1. Bowl of Berry Bliss Smoothie:**

**Ingredients list:**

- One cup of berry mixture (strawberries, blueberries, raspberries).
- One frozen banana
- Half a cup of Greek yogurt
- One-fourth cup of almond milk
- a single spoonful of chia seeds

- One tablespoon of optional maple syrup or honey
- Granola, nut slices, fresh berries, and a honey drizzle serve as toppings.

**Guidelines:**

1. Blend frozen banana, mixed berries, Greek yogurt, almond milk, chia seeds, and honey (if desired) in a blender.
2. Blend until creamy and smooth, adding more almond milk as necessary to modify the consistency.
3. Fill a bowl with the smoothie.
4. Add honey, sliced almonds, fresh berries, and granola over top.
5. Savor your colorful, nutrient-rich Berry Bliss Smoothie Bowl!

**2. Green Goddess Bowl of Smoothies:**

**Ingredients list:**

- one cup of spinach leaves
- A half-ripe avocado
- one-half frozen mango
- Half a cup of chunky pineapple
- Half a cup of coconut water

- One spoonful of rolled oats
- Toppers: Kiwi slices, chia seeds, coconut flakes, and granola sprinkles

## Guidelines:

1. Blend spinach leaves, ripe avocado, frozen mango, pieces of pineapple, coconut water, and flaxseeds together in a blender.
2. Add more coconut water as necessary to alter the consistency after blending until it's smooth and creamy.
3. Transfer the spinach smoothie to a bowl.
4. Add some granola, chia seeds, coconut flakes, and sliced kiwi on top.
5. Savour this hydrating, nutrient-dense Green Goddess Smoothie Bowl!

## 3. Smoothie Bowl with Tropical Paradise:

## Ingredients list:

- one cup of pieces of frozen pineapple
- Half a frozen banana
- Half a cup of chunky mango
- Half a cup of orange juice
- One-fourth cup of coconut milk
- one spoonful of hemp seeds

- Toppers: A handful of oats, shredded coconut, sliced banana, and passion fruit seeds

**Guidelines:**

1. Blend frozen pineapple chunks, frozen banana chunks, frozen mango chunks, orange juice, coconut milk, and hemp seeds using a blender.
2. If necessary, add more orange juice to alter the consistency after blending until it's smooth and creamy.
3. Transfer the exotic drink into a dish.
4. Add some granola, chopped banana, shredded coconut, and passion fruit seeds on top.
5. Savour the unique taste of the Tropical Paradise Smoothie Bowl!

Smoothie bowls are a great way to start the day and promote your overall health, particularly if you have Hashimoto's disease. They're tasty and nutrient-dense.

## Hearty Quinoa Porridge

**Ingredients list:**

- 1/2 cup of washed and drained quinoa

- One cup of almond milk (or any other kind of milk)
- mashed half of a ripe banana
- a single spoonful of chia seeds
- one-half tsp. of ground cinnamon
- One-fourth teaspoon of vanilla essence
- a dash of salt
- Toppers: sliced strawberries, chopped nuts (walnuts and almonds), coconut flakes, honey or maple syrup, and a drizzle

**Guidelines:**

1. If there is a bitter coating on the quinoa, rinse it in cold water.
2. Add the quinoa, almond milk, mashed banana, chia seeds, vanilla essence, cinnamon, and a little amount of salt to a small pot.
3. Put the mixture over medium heat and bring it to a boil. Once boiling, lower the heat to a simmer, cover, and cook the quinoa for 15 to 20 minutes, or until it is tender and has soaked up most of the liquid. Now and again, stir.
4. You may adjust the consistency of the porridge by adding a small amount of extra almond milk if it becomes too thick.
5. Adjust sweetness to taste.

6. After tasting the porridge, adjust the sweetness with honey or maple syrup. You may modify the sweetness to your taste since the ripe banana naturally provides sweetness.
7. Turn off the heat when the quinoa is cooked through and the porridge has thickened. Give it some time to rest—a few minutes.
8. Pour the porridge made of quinoa into bowls and top with your preferred ingredients. A delightful and filling mixture is made with sliced strawberries, chopped almonds, and honey drizzled over.
9. Add other toppings to your porridge if you'd like, such as a handful of fresh berries, a dollop of Greek yogurt, or a sprinkle of flaxseed.
10. Warm up and enjoy your filling quinoa porridge. You'll be full and energized all morning long with this nutritious and filling meal.

A wholesome way to start the day, this hearty quinoa porridge is adaptable and satisfying.

## Nutrient-Packed Breakfast Muffins

## Ingredients list:

- one cup of rolled oats
- One cup of flour, either whole wheat or gluten-free
- half a cup of almond flour
- 1/4 cup of flaxseeds, ground
- One teaspoon of baking powder
- Half a teaspoon of baking soda
- one-half teaspoon of cinnamon
- One-fourth teaspoon of salt
- two mashed, ripe bananas
- Two huge eggs
- One-fourth cup of melted coconut oil
- 1/4 cup of maple syrup or honey
- one tsp vanilla essence
- Half a cup of Greek yogurt or a substitute for dairy
- one-half cup of carrots, grated
- Half a cup of blueberries, either frozen or fresh
- 1/4 cup of chopped nuts, such as pecans, almonds, or walnuts

## Guidelines:

1. Set the oven temperature to 175°C/350°F. Grease the cups or line a muffin tray with paper liners.

2. The ground flaxseeds, whole wheat flour, almond flour, baking powder, baking soda, cinnamon, and salt should all be combined in a big bowl with the rolled oats. Stir well.
3. Mash the ripe bananas with a fork in another bowl until they're smooth.
4. Mix the Greek yogurt, eggs, melted coconut oil, honey, or maple syrup, and vanilla extract with the mashed bananas. Stir until well blended.
5. Fill the bowl with the dry ingredients and then add the liquid ingredients. Just blend by stirring. Steer clear of overmixing.
6. Gently mix the blueberries, chopped almonds, and shredded carrots into the batter.
7. Fill each muffin cup approximately two-thirds full with batter as you spoon it into them.
8. Bake for 18 to 20 minutes, or until a toothpick inserted in the center comes out clean, in a preheated oven.
9. After a few minutes of cooling in the muffin pan, move the muffins to a wire rack to finish cooling.
10. Savour these nutritious breakfast muffins as a quick and delicious morning snack. Any leftovers should be kept refrigerated to maintain freshness.

# Chapter 3

## Lunchtime Fuel

### Vibrant Salad Creations

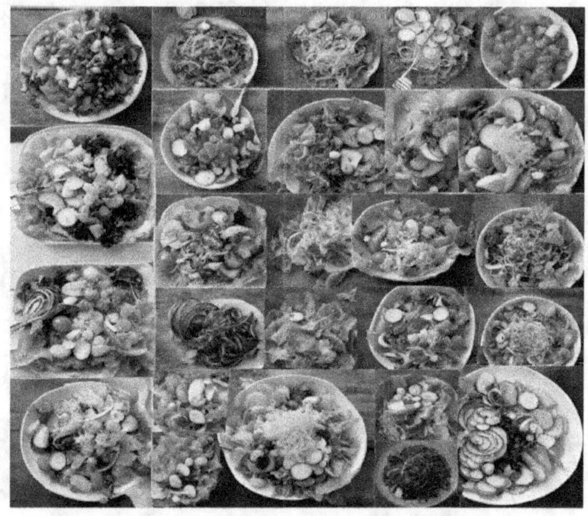

Salads are a canvas for creativity, and these vivid salad concoctions not only pop with color but also give a potent dose of nutrition. Perfect for individuals managing Hashimoto's, these salads are rich in antioxidants, fiber, and important vitamins. Mix and combine items depending on your preferences for a great and healthy dinner.

## 1. Rainbow Quinoa Salad:

**Ingredients**:

- 1 cup cooked quinoa (cooled)
- 1 cup cherry tomatoes, halved 1 cucumber, diced 1 bell pepper (any color), diced 1/2 red onion, finely chopped 1/4 cup feta cheese, crumbled
- Fresh basil and mint leaves, chopped Olive oil, and balsamic vinegar dressing
- Salt and pepper to taste

**Instructions:**

1. In a large bowl, add cooked quinoa, cherry tomatoes, cucumber, bell pepper, red onion, and feta cheese.
2. Toss the salad with chopped basil and mint.
3. Drizzle with olive oil and balsamic vinegar dressing, then season with salt and pepper.
4. Mix well and enjoy this bright and protein-packed quinoa salad.

## 2. Kale and Mango Sunshine Salad:

**Ingredients**:

- 4 cups kale, destemmed and chopped
- 1 ripe mango, peeled and sliced
- 1/4 cup red cabbage, thinly sliced
- 1/4 cup carrots, julienned
- 1/4 cup pumpkin seeds
- Avocado slices for creaminess
- Lemon-tahini dressing
- Salt and pepper to taste

**Instructions:**

1. Massage the chopped kale with a little salt to loosen its texture.
2. In a large bowl, add kale, chopped mango, red cabbage, julienned carrots, and pumpkin seeds.
3. Top the salad with avocado slices.
4. Drizzle with a lemon-tahini dressing and season with salt and pepper.
5. Toss gently and relish the aromas of this nutrient-rich kale and mango salad.


**3. Mediterranean Chickpea Salad:**


**Ingredients:**

- 1 can (15 oz) chickpeas, drained and rinsed

- 1 cup cherry tomatoes, halved 1 cucumber, diced 1/2 red onion, coarsely chopped 1/4 cup Kalamata olives, sliced 1/4 cup crumbled feta cheese
- Fresh parsley, chopped Olive oil, and lemon juice dressing
- Salt and pepper to taste

**Instructions**:

1. In a large bowl, add chickpeas, cherry tomatoes, cucumber, red onion, olives, and feta cheese.
2. Sprinkle fresh parsley over the salad.
3. Drizzle with olive oil and lemon juice dressing, then season with salt and pepper.
4. Toss the salad gently, and appreciate the Mediterranean tastes in every mouthful.
5. Wholesome Soups for Sustained Energy: Nourishing Bowls of Comfort

**4. Lentil and Vegetable Soup:**

**Ingredients:**

- 1 cup dry green or brown lentils, rinsed 1 onion, diced 2 carrots, sliced 2 celery stalks, chopped 3 cloves garlic, minced
- 1 can (14 oz) chopped tomatoes
- 6 cups vegetable broth
- 1 teaspoon ground cumin
- 1 teaspoon smoked paprika
- 1/2 teaspoon turmeric
- Salt and pepper to taste
- Fresh parsley for garnish

**Instructions**:

1. In a large saucepan, sauté the onion, carrots, celery, and garlic until softened.
2. Add lentils, diced tomatoes, vegetable broth, cumin, smoked paprika, turmeric, salt, and pepper.
3. Bring the soup to a boil, then decrease heat and simmer until lentils are cooked (approximately 25-30 minutes).
4. Garnish with fresh parsley before serving.

## 5. Quinoa and Vegetable Minestrone:

**Ingredients**:

- 1/2 cup quinoa, washed

- 1 tablespoon olive oil
- 1 onion, diced 2 carrots, sliced 2 zucchinis, diced 3 cloves garlic, minced 1 can (14 oz) kidney beans, drained and rinsed
- 1 can (14 oz) chopped tomatoes
- 6 cups vegetarian broth 1 teaspoon dried oregano
- 1 teaspoon dried basil
- Salt and pepper to taste
- Fresh basil leaves for garnish

**Instructions:**

1. In a large saucepan, sauté the onion, carrots, zucchini, and garlic in olive oil until the veggies are soft.
2. Add quinoa, kidney beans, chopped tomatoes, vegetable broth, oregano, basil, salt, and pepper.
3. Bring to a boil, then decrease heat and simmer until quinoa is cooked (approximately 15-20 minutes).
4. Garnish with fresh basil leaves before serving.

**6. Coconut Curry Chickpea Soup:**

**Ingredients:**

- 1 tablespoon coconut oil
- 1 onion, diced 2 carrots, sliced 2 bell peppers, diced 3 cloves garlic, minced 1 can (15 oz) chickpeas, drained and rinsed
- 1 can (14 oz) coconut milk
- 4 cups vegetable broth
- 2 teaspoons red curry paste
- 1 teaspoon ground turmeric
- Salt and pepper to taste
- Fresh cilantro for garnish

**Instructions**:

1. In a large saucepan, sauté the onion, carrots, bell peppers, and garlic in coconut oil until softened.
2. Add chickpeas, coconut milk, vegetable broth, red curry paste, turmeric, salt, and pepper.
3. Bring to a simmer and cook for 15-20 minutes.
4. Garnish with fresh cilantro before serving.

## Power-Packed Wraps and Sandwiches

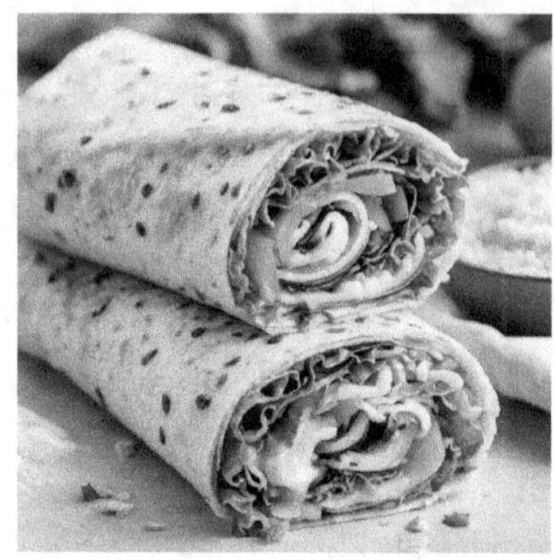

## 1. Spinach and Turkey Avocado Wrap:

### Ingredients list:

- Grain-free or gluten-free wrap
- turkey breast slices
- Cuts of avocado
- new spinach leaves
- slices of tomato
- Hummus on toast
- Mustard Dijon
- Add salt and pepper to taste.

### Guidelines:

1. Spread a layer of Dijon mustard and hummus on the flattened wrap.
2. Place pieces of tomato, avocado, fresh spinach, and turkey on the wrap.

3. Add pepper and salt according to taste.
4. Tightly roll the wrap, cut it in half, and savor this nutrient- and protein-rich treat.

## 2. Vegetable and Chickpea Hummus Wrap:

**Ingredients list:**

- Grain-frcc or gluten-free wrap
- Canary chickpeas, cherry tomatoes, cucumbers, red onions, olives, feta cheese, olive oil, and lemon juice combine to make a salad.
- Hummus on toast
- Arugula fresh
- Lucerne or broccoli sprouts
- Add salt and pepper to taste.

## Guidelines:

1. Put the ingredients for the chickpea salad in a bowl and stir.
2. Spread a thick coating of hummus over the flattened wrapper.
3. Top with sprouts and freshly chopped rocket after spooning the chickpea salad into the wrap.
4. Add pepper and salt according to taste.

5. Enjoy this plant-based masterpiece by rolling the wrap and, if necessary, fastening it with toothpicks.

## 3. Caesar Wrap with Grilled Chicken:

**Ingredients list:**

- Grain-free or gluten-free wrap
- sliced Romaine lettuce and grilled chicken breast
- Grated Caesar dressing, cherry tomatoes, and halved Parmesan cheese
- Whole-grain breadcrumbs (not required)
- Add salt and pepper to taste.

**Guidelines:**

1. Arrange the grilled chicken slices, cherry tomatoes, and Romaine lettuce on a flattened wrap.
2. Over the mixture, scatter the grated Parmesan cheese.
3. Pour over some Caesar dressing and, if preferred, top with whole-grain croutons.
4. Add pepper and salt according to taste.
5. Roll, cut, and enjoy the traditional flavors of a Caesar salad in a portable format.

These nutrient-dense wraps and sandwiches include a balance of fresh veggies, healthy fats, and proteins, which makes them perfect for controlling Hashimoto's

# Chapter 4

## Dinner Delights

### Protein-Packed Main Courses

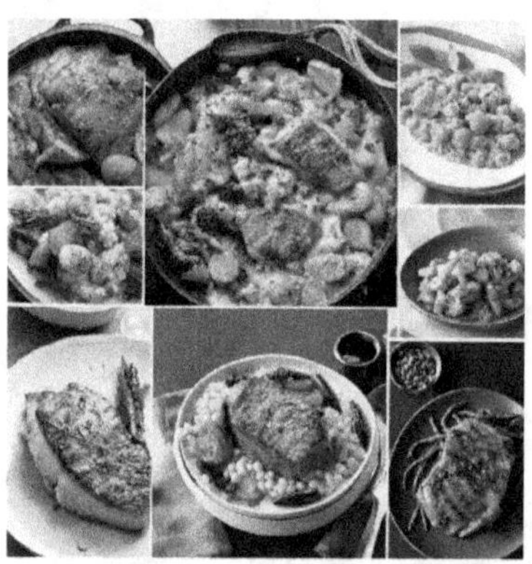

**1. Salmon with Baked Lemon Garlic:**

**Ingredients list:**

- four fillets of salmon
- Two teaspoons of olive oil
- minced three garlic cloves
- One teaspoon of lemon juice and zest
- One tsp. of dried oregano
- Add salt and pepper to taste.
- For garnish, use fresh parsley.

**Guidelines:**

1. heat the oven to 400°F, or 200°C.
2. Salmon fillets should be placed on a parchment paper-lined baking pan.
3. Combine olive oil, minced garlic, lemon zest, lemon juice, dried oregano, salt, and pepper in a small bowl.
4. Salmon fillets should be brushed with the mixture.
5. Salmon should be baked for 12 to 15 minutes, or until it is done.
6. Add some fresh parsley as a garnish and serve with your preferred side dishes.

**2. Stuffed bell peppers with quinoa and black beans:**

**Ingredients list:**

- 4 bell peppers, seeded and cut in half
- 1-cup cooked quinoa
- One fifteen-ounce can of rinsed and drained black beans
- one cup of kernel corn
- one cup of chopped tomatoes
- One cup of cooked, shredded chicken (optional)

- One tsp cumin
- one tsp of chilli powder
- Add salt and pepper to taste.
- Cheese shreds (optional) as a garnish
- For garnish, use fresh cilantro.

**Guidelines:**

1. Set oven temperature to 375°F, or 190°C.
2. Put cooked quinoa, black beans, corn, chopped tomatoes, cumin, chili powder, salt, and pepper in a big bowl. You may also add shredded chicken if you're using it.
3. Place the quinoa mixture into each bell pepper half.
4. Pack the peppers into a baking dish, cover with foil, and bake for twenty to thirty minutes.
5. For the last five minutes of baking, sprinkle some shredded cheese on top if you'd like.
6. Before serving, add some fresh cilantro as a garnish.

**3. Chicken Breast with Grilled Lemon Herb:**

**Ingredients list:**

- 4 skin-and bone-free chicken breasts
- Two teaspoons of olive oil

- one lemon's juice
- minced two garlic cloves
- One tsp. of dried thyme
- one tsp of dried rosemary
- Add salt and pepper to taste.
- Slices of lemon to serve

**Guidelines:**

1. Turn the heat up to medium-high on the grill.
2. Combine olive oil, lemon juice, minced garlic, rosemary dried thyme, salt, and pepper in a bowl.
3. Apply the blend to the chicken breasts.
4. Cook on the grill for 6 to 8 minutes on each side, or until the chicken is done.
5. Accompany with your preferred side dishes with lemon wedges.

These filling, high-protein main dishes complement a healthy, well-balanced diet for people with Hashimoto's by providing a range of flavors and textures.

## Flavorful Grain and Vegetable Bowls

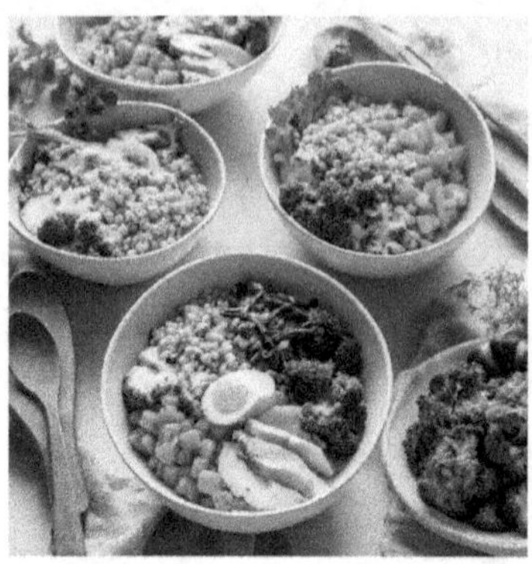

These savory grain and vegetable bowls will elevate your meals; they're not only very tasty but also nutrient-rich for those with Hashimoto's disease. These bowls are a filling and nutritious option since they are full of good grains, colorful veggies, and delectable toppings.

**Quinoa bowl with a Mediterranean flair:**

**Ingredients list:**

- one cup of quinoa, cooked
- Cherry tomatoes,
- cucumbers cut in half,
- chopped Kalamata olives,
- red onion slices,
- finely chopped Feta cheese, crumbled
- chopped parsley,
- lemon juice dressing,

- and olive oil
- Add salt and pepper to taste.

**Guidelines:**

1. Arrange cooked quinoa as the bottom layer in a bowl.
2. Add chopped feta cheese, red onion, cucumber, Kalamata olives, and cherry tomatoes on top.
3. Pour over some lemon juice dressing and olive oil.
4. Add a dash of pepper and salt, and some fresh parsley for garnish.
5. Enjoy this cool dish with a Mediterranean influence after giving it a little toss.

**2. :**

**Ingredients list:**

- one cup of brown rice, cooked
- Cubed, extra-firm tofu cooked with teriyaki sauce
- Steam-cooked broccoli florets,
- carrots,
- red bell pepper (julienned or shredded),
- edamame slices,
- and shelled sesame seeds as garnish

- To drizzle, add chopped Teriyaki sauce and green onions.

## Guidelines:

1. In a bowl, arrange the cooked brown rice.
2. Add the edamame, sliced red bell pepper, steaming broccoli, julienned carrot, and sautéed teriyaki tofu.
3. Top with chopped green onions and sesame seeds.
4. For more flavor, drizzle with more teriyaki sauce.
5. Enjoy this tasty dish full of protein after thorough mixing.

**Black Bean and Southwest Quinoa Bowl:**

**Ingredients list:**

- one cup of quinoa, cooked
- Finely chopped red onion, halved cherry tomatoes, black beans, corn kernels that have been canned and drained, cooked avocado and
- Lime wedges for serving with freshly chopped cilantro
- lime-chipotle dressing
- Add salt and pepper to taste.

## Guidelines:

1. Place cooked quinoa in a bowl to form a foundation.
2. Add the red onion, cherry tomatoes, sliced avocado, cooked corn kernels, and black beans.
3. Add chopped cilantro on the top.
4. Serve with slices of lime on the side.
5. After adding a drizzle of chipotle lime dressing, add salt and pepper to taste.
6. Gently toss and enjoy the flavors of this colorful dish with Southwest influences.

## Oven-Baked Goodness: Casseroles and One-Pan Wonders

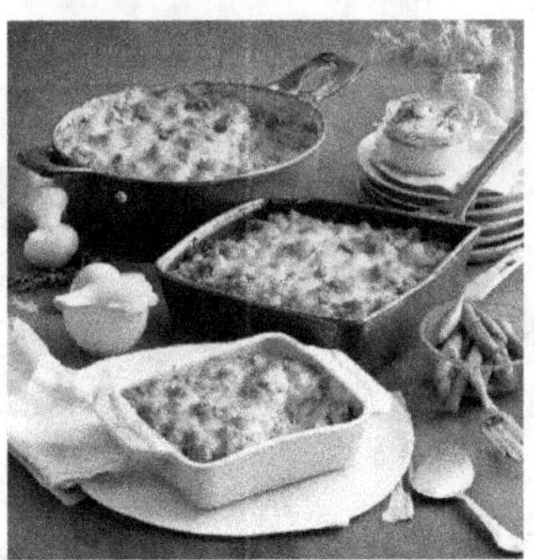

**Quinoa casserole with poultry and vegetables:**

**Ingredients list:**

- Rinse and drain 1 cup of quinoa
- Two cups of shredded cooked chicken
- Two cups of mixed veggies, such as carrots, peas, and broccoli
- One cup of shredded cheddar cheese
- Two cups of broth made from chickens
- 1 cup milk, either non-dairy or dairy
- Two teaspoons of olive oil
- Two tablespoons of all-purpose flour, or a gluten-free substitute
- One tsp powdered garlic
- Add salt and pepper to taste.
- For garnish, use fresh parsley.

**Guidelines**:

1. Set oven temperature to 375°F, or 190°C.
2. Olive oil should be heated in a pan. Add the flour and mix to produce a roux.
3. Whisk continually to prevent lumps as you gradually add the milk and chicken broth.
4. Add some salt, pepper, and garlic powder for flavor. The sauce will thicken after simmering.
5. Put cooked quinoa, mixed veggies, shredded chicken, and half of the cheese in a big bowl.
6. Thoroughly combine the quinoa mixture after adding the sauce.

7. After transferring the mixture to a baking dish and topping it with the remaining cheese, bake it for 25 to 30 minutes, or until brown.
8. Before serving, add some fresh parsley on top.

## 2. Dinner of baked salmon on a sheet pan with vegetables:

**Ingredients list:**

- four fillets of salmon
- Half a pound of baby potatoes
- Broccoli florets in two cups
- Three tablespoons of olive oil, one sliced lemon, and one sliced red bell pepper
- Two tsp of dehydrated thyme
- One tsp powdered garlic
- Add salt and pepper to taste.
- Add some fresh dill as a garnish.

**Guidelines:**

1. heat the oven up to 400°F, or 200°C.

2. Arrange broccoli, red bell pepper, baby potatoes, and salmon fillets on a large baking sheet.
3. Sprinkle salt, pepper, garlic powder, dried thyme, and olive oil over the mixture.
4. To get an even coating, combine everything.
5. Cover the salmon fillets with slices of lemon.
6. Bake the salmon for 20 to 25 minutes, or until it's well done, and the veggies are soft.
7. Before serving, add some fresh dill on top.

## 3. Enchilada casserole with beef and black beans:

**Ingredients list:**

- A single pound of ground beef
- one chopped onion
- one chopped bell pepper
- One fifteen-ounce can of rinsed and drained black beans
- Ten-ounce can of enchilada sauce
- Eight little corn tortillas
- Two cups of Mexican cheese mix, shredded
- One tsp of ground cumin
- one tsp of chilli powder

- Add salt and pepper to taste.
- For garnish, use fresh cilantro.
- sliced avocados to serve

**Guidelines:**

1. Set oven temperature to 375°F, or 190°C.
2. Brown the ground beef in a pan together with the bell pepper and sliced onion. Remove extra fat.
3. Add the ground cumin, chili powder, black beans, enchilada sauce, salt, and pepper. Let it simmer for five minutes.
4. Arrange the meat mixture, shredded cheese, and corn tortillas in a baking dish. Do the same with the other two layers.
5. The cheese should be melted and bubbling after 20 to 25 minutes in the oven.
6. Add some fresh cilantro as a garnish and serve with avocado slices.

For those with Hashimoto's disease, these one-pan meals and oven-baked casseroles provide a tasty and easy way to prepare meals. Savor these dishes' simplicity without sacrificing flavor or nutrition.

# Chapter 5

## Snack Attack

### Guilt-Free Snacking: Nuts, Seeds, and Trail Mixes

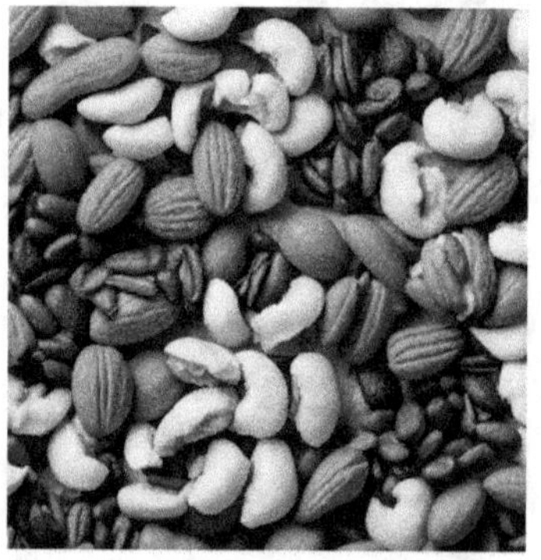

Up the ante on your snack game with guilt-free alternatives that are high in taste and vital nutrients. For those with Hashimoto's disease, trail mixes, nuts, and seeds provide easy and filling snacks. These are a few tasty and filling suggestions:

**1. Almond Energy Bits:**

**Ingredients list:**

- 1 cup mixed nuts, including cashews, walnuts, and almonds
- one-half cup of pitted dates
- Half a cup of chia seeds
- Two teaspoons of coconut shreds without sugar
- One tsp almond butter
- one tsp vanilla essence
- a dash of salt

**Guidelines**:

1. Pulse mixed nuts in a food processor until finely chopped.
2. Include the almond butter, dates, chia seeds, shredded coconut, vanilla essence, and a little amount of salt.
3. Until a sticky dough develops, pulse the ingredients.
4. Form dough into small, bite-sized balls.
5. Chill for a minimum of half an hour before consumption.

**2. Super food Trail Mix:**

**Ingredients list:**

- one cup of almonds
- Half a cup of pumpkin seeds
- Goji berries, half a cup, dry
- 1/4 cup dark chocolate chips with a minimum of 70% cocoa content
- 1/4 cup dried cranberries without added sugar
- One-fourth cup of coconut chips

## Guidelines:

1. Almonds, pumpkin seeds, goji berries, coconut chips, dark chocolate chips, and dried cranberries should all be combined in a dish.
2. After thoroughly mixing, distribute into snack-sized containers.
3. Savor this trail mix on the fly, loaded with superfoods.

## 3. Chickpea Trail Mix Roasted:

## Ingredients list:

- One fifteen-ounce can of washed and drained chickpeas
- A single spoonful of olive oil
- A single tsp of smoky paprika

- one-half teaspoon of cumin
- Half a teaspoon of powdered garlic
- Half a teaspoon of sea salt
- half a cup of uncooked almonds
- 1/2 cup chopped dried apricots
- Pumpkin seeds, or pepitas, 1/4 cup

## Guidelines:

1. heat the oven to 400°F, or 200°C.
2. After using a paper towel to pat dry, put the chickpeas on a baking sheet.
3. Add smoked paprika, cumin, garlic powder, sea salt, and olive oil to the chickpeas and toss.
4. To make it crispy, roast for 20 to 25 minutes.
5. Pepitas, dried apricots, raw almonds, and roasted chickpeas should all be combined in a dish.
6. Chill it before putting it in an airtight container.

## 4. Vanilla-Cinnamon Almond Blend:

## Ingredients list:

- one cup of uncooked almonds

- Melted coconut oil, one tablespoon
- One-third teaspoon maple syrup
- One tsp finely ground cinnamon
- One-half tsp vanilla extract
- a little pinch of sea salt

**Guidelines**:

1. Start the oven to 150°C/300°F.
2. Combine raw almonds, ground cinnamon, maple syrup, melted coconut oil, vanilla essence, and a little amount of sea salt in a bowl.
3. On a baking sheet covered with parchment paper, distribute the almonds.
4. Bake, stirring halfway through, for 20 to 25 minutes.
5. Before putting the almonds in a jar, let them cool.

With their balance of fiber, protein, and healthy fats, these guilt-free snacks are a great option for anybody managing Hashimoto's. Savor them as a handy and wholesome complement to your regular nibbles.

## Savory and Sweet Energy Bites

**1. Savory energy bites with cheese and herbs:**

**Ingredients list:**

- one cup of rolled oats
- Grated Parmesan cheese (1/2 cup) and sunflower seeds (1/2 cup)
- 1½ cups finely chopped fresh parsley and 1/4 cup finely chopped chives.
- One-fourth cup of olive oil
- A single spoonful of Dijon mustard
- One minced garlic clove
- Add salt and pepper to taste.

**Guidelines**:

1. Place rolled oats, Parmesan cheese, sunflower seeds, parsley, and chives in a food processor.
2. Pulse the ingredients until a gritty texture forms.
3. The oat mixture should be combined with olive oil, Dijon mustard, chopped garlic, salt, and pepper in a bowl.
4. Form the batter into small, bite-sized balls.
5. Chill for a minimum of half an hour before serving.

**2. Chocolate Energy Bites with Almonds and Coconut:**

**Ingredients list**:

- one cup of almonds
- Half a cup of unsweetened shredded coconut
- one-fourth cup of cacao powder
- One-fourth cup of almond butter
- 1/4 cup of maple syrup or honey
- one tsp vanilla essence
- a dash of salt
- More coconut shreds for coating

**Guidelines**:

1. Grind almonds to a fine powder in a food processor.
2. Add the almond butter, honey, maple syrup, shredded coconut, vanilla essence, cacao powder, and a dash of salt.
3. Add enough pulses to bring the mixture together.
4. After forming the mixture into bite-sized balls, roll them in more shredded coconut.
5. Chill for a minimum of half an hour before consumption.

**3. Energy Bites with Sun-Dried Tomato and Basil:**

**Ingredients list:**

- One cup of sun-dried tomatoes (not fried in oil), washed and soaked in hot water
- one cup of almonds
- one-fourth cup of fresh basil leaves
- two tsp nutritional yeast
- A single spoonful of olive oil
- one tablespoon of lemon juice
- One garlic clove
- Add salt and pepper to taste.

**Guidelines**:

1. Combine sun-dried tomatoes, almonds, basil, nutritional yeast, olive oil, lemon juice, garlic, salt, and pepper in a food processor and pulse until thoroughly blended.
2. Form the batter into small, bite-sized balls.
3. Chill for a minimum of half an hour before serving.

In addition to being tasty, these savory and sweet energy bites provide a well-rounded combination of nutrients. Adjust the recipes to suit your own tastes and savor these easy-to-make snacks that help you maintain your energy levels while controlling Hashimoto's.

# Dips and Spreads for Tasty Snack Time

## 1. Hummus Duo: Classic and Roasted Red Pepper

### Classic Hummus:

### Ingredients:

- 1 can (15 oz.) washed and drained chickpeas
- 1/4 cup tahini
- 2 tbsp olive oil
- 2 garlic cloves, minced
- 1 tsp cumin
- lemon juice
- Season with salt and pepper to taste
- Water (as required for uniformity)
- Roasted Red Pepper Hummus:
- 1/2 cup roasted red peppers (jarred or handmade)

1. **Instructions:**
2. In a food processor, blend chickpeas, tahini, olive oil, minced garlic, ground cumin, lemon juice, salt, and pepper.
3. Blend until smooth, adding water as required to get the desired consistency.

4. To make Roasted Red Pepper Hummus, add roasted red peppers to the regular hummus and mix until fully integrated.
5. Serve with fresh vegetables, pita, or whole-grain crackers.

## 2. Guacamole with a Twist:

**Ingredients**:

- 3 ripe avocados, peeled and mashed
- 1 tomato, diced
- 14 cup coarsely chopped red onion
- 1 lime, juiced 1 jalapeno, coarsely chopped (optional for heat)
- Season with salt and pepper to taste
- 1/2 teaspoon cumin (optional)

**Instructions:**

1. In a mixing dish, add mashed avocados, diced tomato, chopped red onion, cilantro, lime juice, and jalapeno.
2. Season with salt, pepper, and cumin (if using).
3. Serve with tortilla chips or veggie sticks.

## 3. Greek Yoghurt Tzatziki:

Ingredients:

- 1 cup Greek yoghurt
- 1 cucumber, grated and drained
- 2 garlic cloves, minced
- 1 tablespoon fresh dill, chopped
- 1 tbsp olive oil
- 1 teaspoon lemon juice
- Season with salt and pepper to taste

## Instructions:

1. In a mixing bowl, add Greek yogurt, grated and drained cucumber, minced garlic, chopped dill, olive oil, and lemon juice.
2. Season with salt and pepper to taste.
3. Refrigerate for at least 30 minutes before serving.
4. Serve with pita bread or as a cool dip for vegetables.

## 4. Baba Ganoush:

Ingredients:

- 2 medium eggplants
- 2 tbsp tahini
- 2 garlic cloves, minced
- lemon juice
- 2 tbsp olive oil
- Season with salt and pepper to taste
- For garnish, use fresh parsley.

## Instructions:

1. Preheat the oven to 400°F (200°C).
2. Prick eggplants with a fork and roast until tender (approximately 45-50 minutes).
3. Once the eggplants have cooled, peel them and put the flesh in a food processor.
4. Mix in the tahini, minced garlic, lemon juice, olive oil, salt, and pepper.
5. Blend until smooth.
6. Garnish with fresh parsley and serve with pita or veggie sticks.

## Nutrient-Dense Desserts

## 1. Dark Chocolate Avocado Mousse:

## Ingredients list:

- two ripe avocados
- Half a cup of unsweetened cocoa powder
- 1/4 cup of maple syrup or honey
- one teaspoon vanilla extract
- With a pinch of salt
- Add fresh berries as a garnish.

## Guidelines:

1. In a food processor or blender, combine ripe avocados, chocolate powder, vanilla essence, maple syrup, honey, and a little pinch of salt.
2. Blend until a creamy, smooth consistency is achieved.
3. Before serving, let it sit for at least half an hour to cool.
4. Savor this smooth and delicious chocolate mousse with luscious berries as a garnish.

## 2. Parfait de Seeds Chia:

## Ingredients list:

- a single spoonful of chia seeds
- One cup of plain or almond milk, without added sugar
- Honey or maple syrup, 1 tablespoon

- one-half tsp vanilla extract
- fresh fruit slices (mango, kiwi, and berries)
- The crunch of seeds and nuts

**Guidelines**:

1. In a mixing bowl, mix chia seeds, almond milk, honey, or maple syrup, and vanilla essence.
2. Refrigerate for at least two hours, preferably overnight, to allow the chia seeds to absorb the liquid and form a pudding-like consistency.
3. In serving glasses, arrange pieces of fresh fruit on top of the chia seed pudding.
4. Mix with some nuts and seeds for crunch.
5. Savour this delicious parfait of chia seed pudding cold.

**Banana and oat cookie recipe:**

**Ingredients list:**

- mashed two bananas that are ripe
- A one-pound bag of rolled oats
- One teaspoon almond butter
- A quarter of a cup of chips, dark chocolate
- 1/4 cup of chopped nuts, either walnuts or almonds

- a half-tsp. vanilla essence and a little pinch of cinnamon
- With a pinch of salt

## Guidelines:

1. Set a baking sheet lined with parchment paper and preheat the oven to 350 degrees Fahrenheit (180 degrees Celsius).
2. Blend bananas, rolled oats, almond butter, dark chocolate chips, chopped nuts, cinnamon, vanilla extract, and a little pinch of salt in a mixing bowl.
3. Transfer the mixture in spoonfuls onto the baking sheet that has been preheated.
4. Bake for twelve to fifteen minutes, or until the edges are browned.
5. When ready to serve, let the cookies cool fully.

## 4. Nuts and Berries with Yoghurt Parfait:

## Ingredients list:

- Greek yogurt or an alternative dairy-free product
- blueberries, raspberries, and strawberries together

- Low-sugar or homemade granola is ideal.
- chopped almonds and walnuts
- Pour some honey or maple syrup over it.

**Guidelines:**

1. In a glass or plate, arrange Greek yogurt and assorted berries.
2. Over the granola layer, scatter chopped nuts.
3. Drizzle with honey or maple syrup for a sweet taste.
4. Reapply the layering and finish with a sprinkling of maple or honey syrup.
5. Savor this nutritious and revitalizing yogurt parfait.

These nutrient-dense candies are not only a delicious diversion but also beneficial to your health. To guarantee a tasty and satisfying treat while treating Hashimoto's, feel free to modify these recipes to your preferences and dietary needs.

## Creative and Healthy Baking

**Banana Bread Made using Almond Flour:**

**Ingredients list:**

- three mashed, ripe bananas
- Three of
- One-fourth cup of melted coconut oil
- one tsp vanilla essence
- Two cups of almond flour
- Half a teaspoon of baking soda
- one-half teaspoon of cinnamon
- a little amount of salt
- Optional: chopped almonds or dark chocolate chips

**Guidelines:**

1. Warm up the oven to 350°F (180°C) and coat a loaf pan with oil.
2. Beat eggs, melted coconut oil, vanilla extract, and mashed bananas together in a bowl.
3. Mix baking soda, cinnamon, almond flour, and a small amount of salt in a separate basin.
4. Thoroughly blend the liquid and solid components.
5. Stir in dark chocolate chips or chopped nuts, if preferred.
6. When a toothpick inserted into the loaf pan comes out clean, bake the batter in the pan for 50 to 60 minutes.

7. Let cool completely before slicing the banana bread.

**2. Cookies with Chocolate Chip Quinoa:**

**Ingredients list:**

- 1 cup chilled cooked quinoa
- Half a cup of almond butter
- 1/4 cup of honey or maple syrup
- one egg
- one tsp vanilla essence
- Half a teaspoon of powdered baking soda
- half a cup of chips made with dark chocolate

**Guidelines**:

1. Set a baking sheet lined with parchment paper and preheat the oven to 350°F (180°C).
2. Combine cooked quinoa, almond butter, honey, maple syrup, egg, vanilla extract, and baking powder in a bowl.
3. Stir in the dark chocolate chunks.
4. Drop dough onto the prepared baking sheet with spoonfuls.
5. Bake until the edges become brown, 12 to 15 minutes.

6. When serving, let the cookies cool.

## 3. Brownies with Sweet Potatoes:

**Ingredients list:**

- one cup of sweet potatoes, mashed
- Half a cup of almond butter
- 1/4 cup of honey or maple syrup
- Just one egg
- one tsp vanilla essence
- one-fourth cup of cocoa powder
- Half a teaspoon of baking soda
- a little amount of salt
- Chips or pieces of dark chocolate for the topping

**Guidelines:**

1. Warm up the oven to 350°F (180°C) and coat a brownie pan with oil.
2. Mash sweet potatoes, almond butter, egg, vanilla extract, and maple syrup or honey should all be combined in a basin.
3. Combine cocoa powder, baking soda, and a small amount of salt in a separate basin.
4. Smoothly blend the dry and wet components.

5. After filling the pan, level the top with the batter.
6. Add chips or pieces of dark chocolate on top.
7. Bake for 25 to 30 minutes, or until a toothpick inserted in the center comes out with a few wet crumbs.
8. Before slicing the brownies into squares, let them cool.

## 4. Muffins with berries and muesli:

### Ingredients list:

- Double-cup old-fashioned oats
- One-tsp baking powder
- one-half teaspoon of cinnamon
- Two ripe bananas, mashed; 1/4 teaspoon salt
- Two of
- A single cup of almond milk
- one tsp vanilla essence
- Berries (raspberries and blueberries) combined for the garnish

### Guidelines:

1. Line a muffin tray with paper liners and preheat the oven to 350°F (180°C).

2. Blend the oats in a blender until they resemble flour.
3. Combine the oat flour, cinnamon, baking powder, and salt in a basin.
4. Mash bananas, eggs, almond milk, and vanilla extract should all be combined in a separate dish.
5. Till well combined, combine the dry and wet components.
6. After filling each muffin cup with batter, sprinkle some mixed berries on top.
7. A toothpick inserted into the center should come out clean after 20 to 25 minutes of baking.
8. When ready to serve, let the muffins cool.

A delicious way to indulge in sweets while adding nutrient-dense foods to your diet is with these inventive and healthful baking ideas.

# Chapter 6

## The Healing Cup: Beverages for Balance

### Soothing Herbal Teas

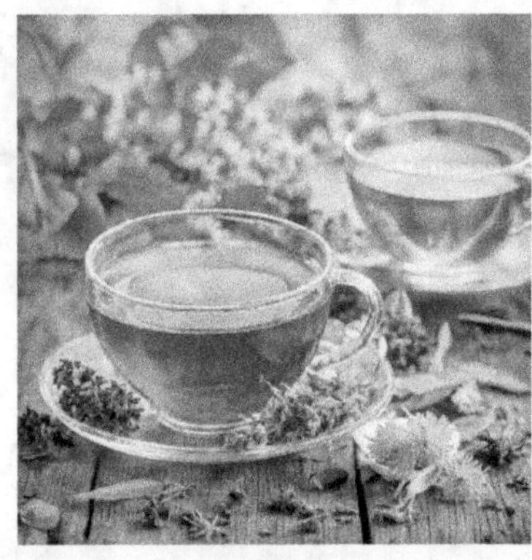

To improve your well-being, especially if you are managing Hashimoto's, embrace the relaxing and restorative qualities of herbal teas. In addition to being tasty, these calming mixes provide a welcome break and may help with immune system support, digestion, and relaxation.

**1. Lavender and Chamomile Tea:**

**Ingredients list:**

- One tea bag of chamomile
- One teaspoon of dried lavender buds
- (Optional) honey
- A slice of lemon, optional

## Guidelines:

1. In boiling water, steep the dried lavender buds and a chamomile tea bag for five to seven minutes.
2. Sift the herbs or take out the teabag.
3. If preferred, add honey for sweetness, and, for added brightness, squeeze in a piece of lemon.
4. Savor the relaxing chamomile and lavender infusion.

## 2. Tea with peppermint and ginger:

**Ingredients list:**

- one bag of peppermint tea
- One teaspoon of shredded fresh ginger with optional honey
- Wedge of lemon, optional

**Guidelines:**

1. In boiling water, steep the peppermint tea bag and freshly grated ginger for five to seven minutes.
2. Take off the tea bag and drain the tea to get rid of any pieces of ginger.
3. If desired, sweeten with honey and add a lemon slice for a tangy touch.
4. Savor the advantages of ginger and peppermint for digestion and refreshment.

**3. Honey tea with lemon balm:**

**Ingredients list:**

- One tea bag with lemon balm.
- One teaspoon of raw honey, with optional lemon zest

**Guidelines**:

1. In boiling water, steep the lemon balm tea bag for five to seven minutes.
2. Until dissolved, stir in raw honey.
3. If you want to add a little more citrus flavor, garnish with lemon zest.
4. Take a sip and enjoy lemon balm's calming effects.

**4. Infusion of Cinnamon and Turmeric:**

**Ingredients list:**

- One teaspoon of either freshly grated turmeric or powder
- One stick of cinnamon
- one teaspoon of honey
- A little pinch of black pepper (to improve the absorption of turmeric).
- Coconut milk—optional

**Guidelines:**

1. Heat some water in a saucepan and add the turmeric, cinnamon stick, and black pepper.
2. Allow the flavors to mingle by simmering for 7 to 10 minutes.
3. Pour out the infusion and mix with the honey.
4. If you want it creamier, add more coconut milk.
5. Savor the warming properties of cinnamon combined with the anti-inflammatory properties of turmeric.

**5. Vanilla Elixir with Rooibos:**

**Ingredients** list:

- One Rooibos tea bag
- One-half teaspoon vanilla extract
- Almond milk (not required)
- Maple syrup (not required)

**Guidelines:**

1. In boiling water, steep the Rooibos tea bag for five to seven minutes.
2. Add the vanilla essence and stir.
3. If you want a creamy texture, add almond milk. If you want to sweeten, use maple syrup.
4. Savor the mild, caffeine-free flavor of rooibos with a touch of vanilla.

## Nutrient-Packed Smoothies

**Smoothie with Green Goddess Detoxification:**

**Ingredients list:**

- One cup of spinach, frozen or fresh
- Half of a cucumber, cut into slices after peeling

- half of an avocado
- half a green apple, cored
- a single spoonful of chia seeds
- Half a lemon's juice
- A single cup of almond milk or coconut water
- Cubes of ice, if desired

**Guidelines**:

1. In a blender, combine spinach, cucumber, avocado, green apple, chia seeds, lemon juice, and almond milk or coconut water.
2. Mix until homogenous.
3. If you want it cooler, add some ice cubes.
4. Enjoy this cooling and cleansing green smoothie after pouring it into a glass.

## 2. Antioxidant Smoothie with Berry Bliss:

**Ingredients list:**

- One cup of berry mixture (strawberries, blueberries, raspberries).
- Half a banana
- Half a cup of Greek or dairy-free yogurt

- One spoonful of rolled oats
- One tsp almond butter
- A single cup of almond milk
- Cubes of ice, if desired

**Guidelines:**

1. Blend mixed berries, almond butter, banana, flaxseeds, Greek yogurt or dairy-free yogurt, and almond milk in a blender.
2. Mix until homogenous.
3. If you want a colder texture, add ice cubes.
4. Pour into a glass and enjoy the berry-packed smoothie's antioxidant-rich deliciousness.

## 3. Sweet Tropical Turmeric:

**Ingredients list:**

- one cup of chunky pineapple
- 1 1/2 mangos, chopped and peeled
- One little banana
- One teaspoonful of freshly grated turmeric or turmeric powder
- a single spoonful of chia seeds
- one cup of coconut water
- Cubes of ice, if desired

**Guidelines**:

1.  Put the pineapple chunks, banana, mango, chia seeds, turmeric, and coconut water in a blender.
2.  Mix until homogenous.
3.  If preferred, add ice cubes.
4.  Transfer into a glass and enjoy the taste of the tropics combined with a hint of anti-inflammatory turmeric.

## 4. Almond Joy Smoothie with Protein Packed:

**Ingredients list:**

- A single cup of almond milk
- Half a cup of Greek or dairy-free yogurt
- One tsp almond butter
- One-third tsp cocoa powder
- One tablespoon of unsweetened coconut shreds
- One scoop of chocolate or vanilla protein powder
- Cubes of ice, if desired

**Guidelines**:

1.  In a blender, combine protein powder, shredded coconut, almond butter, Greek

yogurt or dairy-free yogurt, chocolate powder, and almond milk.

2. Mix until homogenous.
3. If you'd like it cooler, add some ice cubes.
4. Pour the smoothie into a glass and enjoy the decadent flavors of this high-protein Almond Joy.

## Hydration Hacks for Thyroid Support

Having an adequate amount of water in your body is not only important for your general health but also has the potential to help support thyroid function. While you are treating Hashimoto's disease, you should try these hydration hacks to ensure that you are providing your body with the fluids it needs.

**1. An Elixir Made of Lemon Water:**

- ✓ It is recommended that you begin your day with a glass of warm water that has been infused with fresh lemon juice.
- ✓ Lemon is an excellent source of vitamin C, which may be beneficial to the health of the thyroid.

✓ In addition to facilitating digestion, the warmth may be a revitalizing method to get your new day started.

## 2. Infusions made from herbs:

✓ Teas made from herbs, such as peppermint, chamomile, or ginger, that do not include caffeine are recommended.
✓ It is possible for herbal infusions to be calming and to add to your regular fluid intake without having the diuretic impact that is associated with drinks that include caffeine.

## Coconut Water Refresher:

✓ Incorporate coconut water into your hydration regimen.
✓ Coconut water is a natural electrolyte-rich beverage that may assist in maintaining adequate hydration levels.

## 4. Hydrating Smoothies:

✓ Make smoothies using hydrating fruits like watermelon, cucumber, and berries.
✓ Blend with a foundation of coconut water or almond milk for an added hydration boost.

## 5. Electrolyte-Rich Drinks:

- ✓ Include liquids that provide important electrolytes, such as potassium and sodium.
- ✓ Coconut water, sports drinks, or a homemade electrolyte drink may help restore electrolytes lost via perspiration.

## 6. Hydration Tracking:

- ✓ Use a water bottle with markers to monitor your water consumption throughout the day.
- ✓ Set hydration goals and try for a regular intake to be well hydrated.

## 7. Infused Water Creations:

- ✓ Enhance your water with natural tastes by infusing it with fruits, herbs, or cucumber slices.
- ✓ Experiment with combos like mint and lime or berries and basil for a delightful twist.

## 8. Broth & Soups:

- ✓ Include hydrating items in your diet, such as clear broths and soups.
- ✓ These may add to your total fluid intake while delivering nutrients.

## 9. Hydration Reminder Apps:

- ✓ Use smartphone applications or alarms to remind you to drink water frequently.

✓ These reminders might help develop a regular hydration practice.

## 10. Salty Snacks in Moderation:

✓ Enjoy salty foods in moderation, since sodium is a necessary electrolyte.
✓ Opt for healthy choices like almonds or seeds to balance water and salt levels.

Remember that individual hydration requirements might vary, therefore it's crucial to listen to your body.

# Beyond the Plate: Lifestyle Tips

## Stress Management Techniques

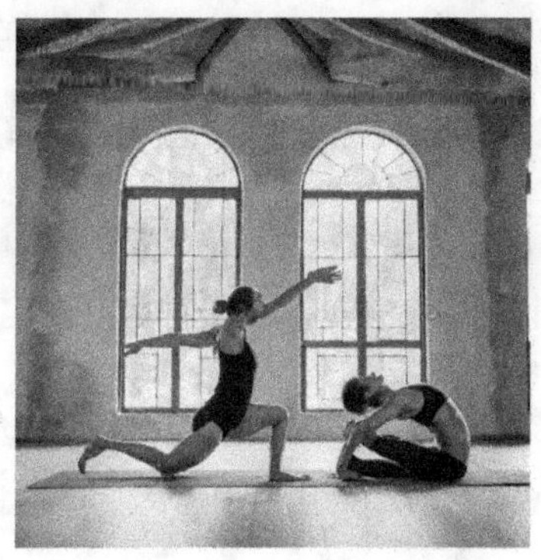

Incorporate these strategies into your daily routine to produce a feeling of tranquility and improve general well-being.

### 1. Mindful Breathing:

- Practice deep breathing techniques to soothe the nervous system.
- Inhale deeply with your nose, hold for a few seconds, then exhale slowly through your mouth.

- Repeat for a few minutes, concentrating on the rhythm of your breath.

## 2. Meditation:

- Set aside time each day for meditation.
- Use guided meditation applications or just locate a quiet spot to concentrate on your breath, a mantra, or peaceful imagery.

## 3. Progressive Muscle Relaxation (PMR):

- Tense and then gradually relax each muscle group in your body, beginning from your toes and working your way up to your head.
- This approach promotes bodily relaxation, relieving tension.

## 4. Yoga and stretching:

- Engage in mild yoga or stretching techniques to alleviate bodily stress.
- Yoga integrates movement with breath, improving both physical and mental well-being.

## 5. Nature Walks:

- Spend time in nature, whether it's a park, a walk, or a garden.
- Connect with the outdoors to alleviate stress and enhance a feeling of tranquility.

## 6. Journaling:

- Pen down your thoughts and emotions in a journal.
- Reflecting on your experiences might bring clarity and help you recognize stress.

## 7. Establishing Boundaries:

- Learn to say no when required.
- Set reasonable limitations on your obligations to avoid overload.

## 8. Positive Affirmations:

- Use positive affirmations to fight negative thinking.
- Repeat affirmations that connect with you to build a good mentality.

## 9. Social Support:

- Connect with friends, family, or support groups.
- Sharing your emotions with others might give emotional support.

## 10. Time Management:

- Prioritize projects and split them into manageable stages.

- Avoid crowding your calendar, and make time for self-care.

## 11. Art and Creativity:

- Engage in creative pursuits like painting, sketching, or making.
- Expressing oneself via art may be soothing.

## 12. Laughter Therapy:

- Watch a hilarious movie, attend a comedy concert, or spend time with individuals who make you laugh.
- Laughter increases the production of endorphins, fostering a happy mood.

## 13. Mindfulness Practices:

- Practice being present in the moment via mindfulness.
- Mindful eating, walking, or just paying attention to your environment might help alleviate stress.

## 14. Massage or self-massage:

- Treat yourself to a massage or discover self-massage methods.

- Massage promotes relaxation and helps eliminate physical strain.

**15. Professional Support:**

- Seek help from mental health specialists when required.
- Therapy or counseling may provide skills and techniques for dealing with stress.

Remember that managing stress is a continuous process, and discovering what works best for you may require a mix of these strategies. Consistency and self-compassion are crucial aspects of building a stress management program that promotes your well-being while treating Hashimoto's or other health concerns.

## Exercise and Movement for Thyroid Health

**1. Cardiovascular Exercise:**

- Engage in aerobic exercises like brisk walking, running, cycling, or swimming.
- Aim for at least 150 minutes of moderate-intensity or 75 minutes of vigorous-intensity aerobic activity every week.

## 2. Strength Training:

- Include resistance or strength training workouts at least two days a week.
- Focus on key muscle groups by utilizing bodyweight workouts, free weights, or resistance bands.

## 3. Yoga:

- Practice yoga to enhance flexibility, balance, and relaxation.
- Certain yoga postures and sequences may directly target the thyroid and increase its function.

## 4. Pilates:

- Incorporate Pilates into your regimen to strengthen the core and enhance total body strength.
- Pilates movements may be tailored to different fitness levels.

## 5. High-Intensity Interval Training (HIIT):

- Consider combining HIIT exercises for brief bursts of intense activity followed by intervals of recuperation.
- HIIT may be useful for improving cardiovascular health and metabolism.

## 6. Walking or Hiking:

- Take advantage of the simplicity and accessibility of walking.
- Regular walks or excursions in nature may be both restorative and good for thyroid health.

## 7. Dancing:

- Enjoy dancing as a pleasant and interesting form of fitness.
- Whether attending dance lessons or dancing at home, it's a terrific method to increase happiness and health.

## 8. Tai Chi:

- Explore the gentle motions of Tai Chi for stress relief and enhanced balance.
- Tai Chi may be a focused and low-impact workout ideal for varied fitness levels.

## 9. Swimming:

- Incorporate swimming as a full-body exercise that is gentle on the joints.
- Swimming may boost cardiovascular fitness and muscle endurance.

## 10. Biking:

- Ride a bicycle for a low-impact, cardiovascular workout.
- Choose relaxing rides or more demanding routes, depending on your fitness level.

## 11. Functional Training:

- Include workouts that mirror daily motions to increase functioning.
- Functional training promotes coordination and strengthens muscles utilized in everyday tasks.

## 12. Mindful Movement:

- Practice mindful movement forms like Qigong to mix mild exercise with awareness.
- These routines may aid in stress reduction and general well-being.

## 13. Group Classes:

- Join group workout programs for motivation and social involvement.
- Whether it's Zumba, spinning, or group exercise, discover what gives you pleasure.

## 14. Stretching:

- Prioritize flexibility with stretching exercises.

- Stretching helps enhance joint range of motion and avoid stiffness.

## 15. Listen to Your Body:

- Pay attention to how your body reacts to exercise.
- Adjust the intensity and length depending on your energy levels and general health.

Before beginning any new workout regimen, particularly if you have underlying health concerns like Hashimoto's, it's essential to check with a healthcare practitioner or fitness specialist. They may give counsel suited to your unique requirements and assist in designing a safe and effective fitness plan to promote thyroid health.

## Sleep Hygiene for Restorative Nights

A good night's sleep is vital for general well-being, especially while treating illnesses like Hashimoto's. Adopt these sleep hygiene techniques to boost the quality of your sleep and support your overall health.

## 1. Consistent Sleep Schedule:

Aim for a regular sleep habit by going to bed and getting up at the same time every day, including on weekends.

Regular sleep patterns assist in regulating your body's internal clock.

## 2. Create a relaxing bedtime routine:

Establish peaceful pre-sleep habits, such as reading a book, performing moderate yoga, or taking a warm bath.

Engage in activities that communicate to your body that it's time to wind down.

## 3. Optimal Sleep Environment:

Keep your bedroom cold, dark, and quiet.

Invest in blackout curtains and comfy bedding, and consider using earplugs or a white noise machine if required.

## 4. Limit screen time before bed.

Reduce exposure to screens at least an hour before sleep.

The blue light released by electronic gadgets may interfere with the generation of the sleep-inducing hormone melatonin.

**5. Mindful Nutrition:**

Avoid large meals close to sleep.

Limit coffee and nicotine consumption, since these may disturb sleep patterns.

**6. Regular physical activity:**

Engage in regular physical activity, but avoid severe exercise close to sleep.

Regular exercise helps improve sleep, but timing is essential.

**7. Manage stress:**

Practice stress-reducing strategies like meditation, deep breathing, or progressive muscle relaxation.

Managing stress may help relax the mind and prepare the body for healthy sleep.

**8. Comfortable Sleep Environment:**

Invest in a comfy mattress and pillows.

Ensure your sleep environment fosters relaxation and promotes a pleasant night.

**9. Limit Naps:**

If you need to nap, keep it brief (20-30 minutes) and early in the day to prevent interfering with evening sleep.

## 10. Be Mindful of Liquid Intake:

Limit beverages close to sleep to lessen the probability of waking up for bathroom excursions.

## 11. Manage Lighting:

Expose oneself to natural light throughout the day to regulate your circadian cycle.

Dim the lights in the evening to indicate to your body that it's time to wind down.

## 12. Address Sleep Disorders:

If you suspect a sleep condition, such as sleep apnea or insomnia, get professional treatment for diagnosis and management.

## 13. Create a Sleep-Conducive Atmosphere:

Keep the bedroom neat and clutter-free.

A well-organized area adds to a more relaxing sleep environment.

## 14. Limit Clock Watching:

Avoid repeatedly checking the clock if you wake up throughout the night.

This might heighten anxiety and make it more difficult to go back to sleep.

**15. Consult with Healthcare Professionals:**

If sleep issues continue, contact a healthcare expert, such as a sleep specialist or your general care physician.

They may provide specialized guidance and actions depending on your unique requirements.

## Dining Out with Hashimoto's

### 1. Plan Ahead:

Check the restaurant's menu online beforehand.

Look for solutions that correspond with your nutritional requirements and tastes.

### 2. Choose Thyroid-Friendly Foods:

Prioritize lean proteins, such as grilled chicken, fish, or plant-based proteins.

Opt for healthful grains, such as quinoa or brown rice, over-processed grains.

### 3. Mindful Carbohydrate Choices:

Be cautious of carbohydrate choices to ensure stable blood sugar levels.

Select complex carbs like sweet potatoes or whole-grain choices.

### 4. Opt for Vegetables:

Embrace a range of bright veggies to increase nutritional intake.

Consider salads, vegetable sides, or grilled veggie platters.

### 5. Watch Portion Sizes:

Be aware of portion proportions, since larger servings might lead to overeating.

Consider splitting meals or asking for a half serving if available.

### 6. Be Sauce Savvy:

Request sauces and dressings on the side.

This provides you control over the quantity you eat, particularly if some elements may not correspond with your nutritional habits.

### 7. Mind the Salt:

Limit additional salt by picking recipes with fewer processed components.

Ask for meals to be cooked with reduced salt if feasible.

### 8. Choose Healthy Fats:

Opt for recipes that feature healthy fats, such as olive oil, avocados, or almonds.

These fats may help to general well-being.

### 9. Inquire About Preparation Methods:

Don't hesitate to inquire about how things are made.

Choose grilled, steamed, or baked selections over fried or excessively processed ones.

### 10. Communicate Dietary Restrictions:

Inform your server about any dietary limitations or preferences.

Most restaurants are eager to fulfill unusual orders when feasible.

### 11. Hydrate Wisely:

Choose water, herbal teas, or other low-sugar drinks.

Limit sugary beverages and excessive caffeine, particularly later in the day.

### 12. Listen to Your Body:

Pay attention to hunger and fullness signals.

Quit eating when you are satisfied to prevent overeating.

### 13. Be Cautious with Allergens:

If you have food allergies, tell them openly to restaurant workers.

Ask about possible cross-contamination issues.

### 14. Bring Your Own Dressing or Sauce:

Consider bringing your own thyroid-friendly dressing or sauce.

This guarantees you have a tasty alternative that corresponds with your nutritional goals.

### 15. Choose Desserts Mindfully:

If indulging in dessert, aim for fruit-based selections or ones with less processed sugars.

Share sweets to savor a taste without overindulging.

Navigating restaurant menus with Hashimoto's needs attention and conversation. By making educated decisions and being proactive about your nutritional requirements, you may enjoy eating out while maintaining your thyroid health. If confused about certain ingredients or cooking techniques, don't hesitate to ask your server for clarification.

## Sharing Your Dietary Needs with Others

When treating Hashimoto's or other dietary restrictions, effective communication is vital to ensure your demands are recognized and respected. Here are some recommendations for discussing your dietary preferences with others:

### 1. Be Confident:

- Approach talks about your nutritional requirements with confidence.
- Remember that your health is a priority, and expressing your wants is a legitimate and vital component of self-care.

### 2. Educate Others:

- Take the opportunity to educate friends, relatives, or coworkers about Hashimoto's and your unique dietary needs.
- Provide them with resources or knowledge to increase their comprehension.

### 3. Choose the Right Time:

- Select an acceptable moment to address your dietary requirements, ensuring that you have the attention of the individuals you are speaking to.
- Avoid bringing up the issue at a busy or distracting time.

### 4. Use "I" Statements:

- Frame your conversation using "I" phrases to explain your demands without appearing accusing.
- For instance, state, "I need to avoid gluten due to my health situation" instead of "You need to accommodate my diet."

### 5. Be Specific:

- Clearly state your dietary limits and preferences.
- Specify certain items to avoid or include and explain any cross-contamination issues.

### 6. Offer Solutions:

- Suggest alternatives or adaptations that make it simpler for others to suit your demands.
- For instance, consider bringing a meal to contribute to a party that corresponds with your dietary preferences.

## 7. Keep it Positive:

- Maintain a pleasant tone while addressing your nutritional demands.
- Emphasize the range of meals you can enjoy rather than concentrating primarily on limits.

## 8. Share Your Motivation:

- Share the health advantages or improvements you've noticed by keeping to your food limitations.
- Connecting your decisions to good results might help others realize the value.

## 9. Be Open to Questions:

- Encourage inquiry and curiosity.
- Offering information and responding to queries may develop understanding and support.

## 10. Express Gratitude:

- Acknowledge and show thanks when people make an effort to meet your dietary preferences.
- Appreciating their assistance promotes a happy and collaborative atmosphere.

## 11. Utilize Technology:

- Leverage technology to your advantage. Share articles, recipes, or applications that may help others understand your nutritional requirements better.

## 12. Plan Ahead:

- When attending gatherings, contact the host ahead of time about your dietary preferences.
- This proactive approach enables simpler planning and consideration.

## 13. Reiterate as Needed:

- Remind friends and family of your dietary preferences, particularly if it's a new change.
- Consistent communication helps cement comprehension.

## 14. Be Flexible:

- Be open to compromise and flexibility when needed.

- While it's crucial to advocate for your health, being adaptive may make social settings more pleasant for everyone.

## 15. Celebrate Your Choices:

- Frame your eating decisions as a positive component of your life.
- Celebrate the healthful meals you choose to include, establishing a positive and inclusive mindset.

# Closing Thoughts

## Celebrating Progress and Small Wins

1. The Mosaic of Growth: Imagine your life as a gorgeous mosaic, each modest victory adding a colorful tile to the masterpiece. Every finished job, every step toward a goal, generates a distinct tint that improves the overall image of your accomplishments.

2. The Symphony of Effort: Picture the trip as a symphony where each modest victory is a note, resonating with the melody of your attempts. From the delicate plucking of strings to the booming pounding of drums, every stride forward contributes its particular sound to the symphony of development.

3. Illuminating the road: Celebrating accomplishment is analogous to hanging lamps along your road. These modest successes brighten the road ahead, throwing a pleasant glow on the following stages of your trip. Each flickering light

communicates, "You're on the right track; keep moving."

4. The Quilt of Resilience: Envision your resilience as a quilt, with every modest victory knitting together the fabric of your inner strength. Whether you conquer a fear, overcome a hurdle, or just stand up for yourself, each thread strengthens the quilt that blankets you in bravery.

5. Dancing with appreciation: Picture appreciation as a dance, and each tiny triumph as a beautiful stride. With every motion, you show gratitude for the progress accomplished, creating a dance of pleasure and thanks that celebrates the beauty of the present moment.

6. Blooming Gardens of Self-Esteem: Imagine your self-esteem as a blooming garden. Each modest triumph is a bud that unfurls into a bright flower, adding not only beauty but also the smell of achievement to the landscape of your self-worth.

7. Echoes of optimism: Envision the waves of optimism that emanate from each modest triumph. Like a pebble thrown into a quiet pond, these successes send forth waves of optimism that impact not just your life but also the lives of people around you.

8. Building Bridges of Confidence: Picture your confidence as a bridge, cemented with the bricks of tiny triumphs. With every success, you reinforce this bridge, enabling you to pass over hurdles and uncertainties with a renewed feeling of security.

9. The Symphony of Grind: Imagine the rhythm of your daily grind as a symphony and each modest triumph as a crescendo in the melody of your efforts. These moments interrupt the melody of your hard work, reminding you of the beauty hidden in your commitment.

10. Constellations of Accomplishments: Envision your successes as stars in the night sky. Each modest success helps to construct constellations that depict the tale of your journey—a cosmic map of your progress.

## Continuing Your Journey to Thyroid Wellness

As you stand at the threshold of continued discovery and well-being on your journey to thyroid health, let these parting words be a gentle breeze, nudging you forward with resilience and hope.

Your path to thyroid wellness is not a destination but an ever-unfolding narrative—a story written with each mindful choice, nourishing meal, and act of self-care. As you continue this journey, remember that it's adorned with both the sunlit meadows of triumph and the shadows of challenges.

In the tapestry of managing Hashimoto's or any thyroid-related condition, the threads of progress are woven with persistence, understanding, and self-compassion. Celebrate the small victories, for they are the heartbeat of your journey—a rhythm that echoes your strength and resilience.

Let the lessons learned be stepping stones, not heavy burdens. Embrace the wisdom gained from setbacks, for they are the compass guiding you towards a stronger, more resilient version of yourself.

As you navigate the nuances of dining out, exercise, sleep hygiene, and sharing your dietary needs, may you find joy in the rituals of self-care and in the knowledge that you are crafting a life infused with well-being.

Remember, the pursuit of thyroid wellness is not a solitary endeavor. Lean on the support of those who surround you—friends, family, healthcare professionals. Their presence is a comforting melody in the symphony of your journey.

Continue to be your own advocate, gently but firmly steering your course towards health and vitality. And when the path seems daunting, when the road feels long, draw strength from the mosaic of progress you've created, where each small win adds a sparkle to your story.

May your days be filled with nourishing foods, joyful movement, restful nights, and moments of grace. May the whispers of self-compassion be a constant companion, and may your journey be adorned with the vibrant hues of well-being.

So, with gratitude for the steps taken and anticipation for the steps yet to come, continue your journey to thyroid wellness. The pages of your story are still being written, and each chapter unfolds with the promise of growth, healing, and a life beautifully lived.\

Wishing you a journey infused with grace, courage, and the radiant glow of thyroid wellness. Onward, dear traveler, toward the horizon of well-being that awaits you.

# Index

## A



## B



## C



## D



## E